5 WAYS TO IMPROVE YOUR
GOLF GAME

Learn to Swing, Drive and Putt Without Pain

Klaus Jørgensen
Physiotherapist

http://www.plus40golf.com

5 WAYS TO IMPROVE YOUR
GOLF GAME
Learn to Swing, Drive and Putt Without Pain

By Klaus Jørgensen

Juviva Group
Klaus Jørgensen
http://www.plus40golf.com
© Copyright Klaus Jørgensen 2016

Table of Contents

"The purpose with this book is to present some practical ideas about personal golf conditioning fitness program that will improve your golf game."

Kind regards
Klaus Jørgensen

The Golf Paradox: How Most Golfers Could Improve Their Golf and How to Do It

At age 19 I was invited to a golf club in San Francisco Bay area. The reason I was at the golf club was to try playing golf for the first time ever in my life. In my mind this was going to be easy. All my life I had been really good at sports, so I though this would be a walk over. Boy was I wrong.

At the driving Range I went at it with confidence. And sure enough my first attempt was the most perfectly executed golf swing ever seen in the history of mankind. That is…until I looked at the ground. The golf ball had not moved at all. That turned out to be one of the most challenging and frustrating days ever for my ego.

"Golf is deceptively simple and endlessly complicated."
Arnold Palmer

That day I decided that golf would never be my game. But little did I realize that 10 years later golf would come into my life again. Now as a physiotherapist with more than 12 years experience in the Health and Wellness industry and 50.000 consultations, I have come across the golf paradox.

And the paradox? On one side we have the golf swing - considered by many as one of the most unnatural, complex and explosive movement in sports. The Golf swing is really demanding and places some of the highest spinal loads.

On the other side of the Golf paradox we have a huge group of uncon-ditioned golfer over 40 how suffers from easy-chair atrophy, creeping obesity, decreasing mobility, stability and power.

Imagine a 10-handicap golfer who takes about 50 hard swings and another 50-75 practice swings and walks about 8000 yards per round. That is a lot of compressive forces, lateral bending and rotational forces on the back.

The average golfer is investing significantly more money on new golf equipment and apparel as to improve his own physical condition. Here, the personal fitness level has a much greater impact on stroke technique and width than the equipment.

The golf season is right around the corner and you are probably well prepared to participate in every golf area but one. That is the area of physical conditioning. It is likely the most important aspect of your preseason preparation. A lot of research studies have been done with senior golfers that significantly improved their health, fitness and driving power for a much better golf game. Perhaps the most important finding has been that the previously injured and injury prone golfers who completes golf-conditioning programs plays essentially pain-free the following season.

A properly trained body avoids complaints, develops more momentum and thus a higher clubhead speed. The body also fatigues slower and you as a player plays at a high level longer.

Results of the exercise shows the potential for improvement which golfers can achieve through mobility, stability and strength training.

Specific training of back muscles should be standard with golfers of all levels.

Top 10 Most Common Golf Injuries

Experts in sports medicine describes a number of possible reasons to common golf swing injuries. They are as follows:

• Overuse and overpractise

• Poor swing mechanics

• Over-swinging

• Not warming up the body properly

• Rotational stresses placed on the spine

• Incorrect grip and setup

• Traumatic force to the body resulting from a poorly executed swing

Back Pain

According to medical statistics 80% of the German population suffer at least once in their lives from back problems. 70-80% of all back problems correlate with weak muscles and stiff joints. Sports Medical studies shows that golfers experience even greater spinal strain. A quarter of all golfers begin a round of golf with mild to significant back pain. Specific studies with golfers clearly show that an isolated training of the spinal muscles caused a significant improvement in the handicap, with a simultaneous decrease of back problems.

Tendinitis in the Elbows

Tendinitis (irritation and inflammation of the tendon tissue) is the most common condition affecting the elbow. It is frequently referred to as "tennis elbow" where there is an injury to the outer tendon, and "golfer's" elbow" when there is an injury to the inner tendon. Interestingly enough, most golfers suffer more from "tennis elbow" than "golfer's elbow".

Knee Pain

Knee pain can occur from the strain placed on a weak knee to stabilize the rotation of the hip axis at the beginning of the swing. Extreme force placed on the knee can result in torn ligaments. Arthritis sufferers may experience more knee problems because the degenerative nature of the disease, which results in a gradual wearing away of joint cartilage.

Shoulder Pain

Pain may be felt in the shoulder or upper arm at various phases of the golf swing, or following play, often during the night and when extending arms overhead. Injuries to the shoulder can be sustained through traumatic force resulting from a poorly executed golf swing, hitting a root or rock, taking a deep divot, and from overuse. Golfers can develop tendinitis, bursitis, and tears in the rotator cuff due to the repetitive motion of the golf swing.

Wrist Injuries

The repetitive motions of golf, and the high speed of the typical swing can place wrists at a high risk for injury. Pain and tenderness on the top of the wrist, experienced at the top of the backswing and at impact, are common. The most common golf-related wrist injury is tendinitis, or swelling of the tendons responsible for wrist movement. Many wrist injuries, as well as other golf-related injuries, can be prevented by a pre-season and year-round golf-specific conditioning program.

Hand and Finger Injuries

Much as with wrist injuries, the repetitive motions of golf, and the high speed of the typical swing can place the hands and fingers at high risk for injury. Repetitive blunt trauma or single severe trauma to the fingers can lead to numerous conditions such as tendinitis, broken or deformed bones.

Neck and Upper Back Injuries

Neck and upper back injuries are common in golfers because of the twisting natur of the golf swing. After a few hours of swinging the club and hitting balls, the neck and upper back muscles may shorten in spasm and freeze the neck into a painful position.

Foot and Ankle Injuries

Throughout the golf swing, the body acts as a whip; power production starts with the feet pushing against the ground. Each foot moves differently during a golf swing. The back foot must allow for more pronation during the follow- through of the golf swing than the front foot. Injuries can occur when the golfer looses his or her footing or balance during the swing, while performing the swing with the improper swing mechanics, and when hitting a ball off an uneven surface.

Hip Injuries

The hip joint is usually very mobile and able to withstand large amounts of loading stresses, but is particularly vulnerable to injury during golf, since the swing involves a tremendous amount of pivoting and twisting movements. During the golf swing, the hip is subjected to repeated adduction and flexion/extension forces. This requires a great deal of control throughout the gluteal muscles and the adductor muscle complex. It is these rotational and shear forces that cause injuries such as groin strains and low back injuries.

Injury to the Ego

EGO. What is it? It's your small self, trying to be big. More often than not, the ego is running the show. The first thing you need to know about your ego: it does not always have your best interest in mind. All the ego wants is to be heard! Like a small child, the ego thrives when you are paying attention to it. It whispers in your ear all day, and sometimes becomes very loud. Golf will destroy your ego evertime.

Learn More About the 10 Most Common Golf Injuries

Learn about how to treat your back, elbow, knees, shoulder, wrist, hand & fingers, neck, upper back, foot & ankle and hips in my online video training course.

http://www.plus40golf.com

---

5 Areas All Golfers Over Forty Need to Address to Improve Their Game and Life

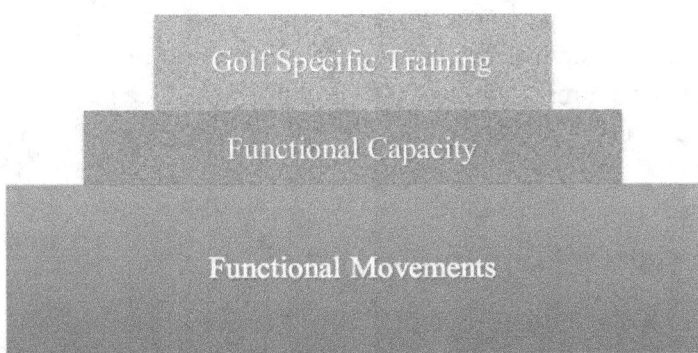

Above you see the Performance Pyramid.

The first level shows the foundation: Functional movements are made up by mobility and stability. Functional movement is the ability to move through fundamental patterns.

The second level shows the functional capacity. Or also called performance. Performance is all about how efficient the body works. How efficient the body produces power. Not specific golf related power, but general power. You can test this with the Vertical leap test.

The third level shows golf specific skills. This level looks at competition statistics and any specific testing relative to golf.

A More Balanced Golfer is a Better Golfer

Most golfers knows more about the latest golf-club than they know about the own bodies and how it works. You as a golfer should try to place yourself and the way your body performance within the performance pyramid to find possible weak links in your golf performance.

There are four basic profiles of the performance pyramid. The optimum performance pyramid, the overpowered performance pyramid, the underpowered performance pyramid and the underskilled performance pyramid.

The Optimum Golf Performance Pyramid

In this golfers pyramid there is a perfect balance between movement patterns, movement efficiency and golf skills. This does not mean that you can not improve, but any improvement should not upset the balance and appearance of the pyramid. This golfer could benefit from improving all three levels, but without sacrificing the balance between the three levels of performance.

The Overpowered Golf Performance Pyramid

In this golfers pyramid the golfer lack a mobility and stability (the first level). But the golfer is able to produce a lot of power and have adequate skills (the third level). This golfer needs to improve movements patterns, but without loosing power.

The Underpowered Golf Performance Pyramid

In this pyramid the golfer has good mobility and good stability (the first level). But lacks gross athleticism or the ability to produce power in simple movements patterns (the second level). This golfer would benefit from power training like strength training.

The Underskilled Golf Performance Pyramid

Now who doesn't belong to this category? In this pyramid the golfer has an optimal functional movement level and an optimal functional performance level. But less than optimal golf skills. This golfer would benefit from golf technique training to improve his or hers game.

Imagine you woke up this morning feeling, stronger than ever, leaner than ever, with a mobile body, perfect stability, coordination and endurance feeling you could handle anything.

Imagine standing on the golf course ready to beat your friends, colleagues or business partners for good with a strong, lean and healthy body...hitting longer and score better.

But... If you are like most golfers you have the best of the best equipment, have invested a lot of money in the right instructors but have not invested much money or time in building a strong, lean and healthy body that can withstand the high forces that are produced by one of the most complex, explosive and physically demanding action - The golf swing.

If you and your body are not in great condition it will affect your playing ability and increase the risk for injuries.

I'm going to show you how to maximize your physical abilities. Your body needs more muscle and less fat. The good news is that you are never too out of shape to start a conditioning program of proper exercise and nutrition.

I will show you that everything you need to get started probably is at your house already. In fact, you won't have to go to a gym at all. And the time spend doing the exercise programs will be minimal.

Imagine all the fitness equipment in a normal fitness club. It looks good and probably feels good, but did you realize that you have the best equipment in the world where you are sitting now? Your own body. Sure you can build and maintain a strong, lean and healthy body that performs great on the golf course, with expensive equipment, but you can build and maintain a strong, lean and healthy body training at your home, the hotel or even on the golf course using your imagination and your own body.

But first here are five reasons your golf game and your life probably is not like you want it to be if you are older than 40.

Easy Chair-Atrophy

As you age you will lose muscle and get weaker. You will actually lose 1/2 a pound of muscles per year between the ages 20 to 50 if you do not engage in regular strength-conditioning programs . At age 50 you will have lost about 15 pounds of muscles compared with the amount of muscles you had when you were 20 years of age.

The reason for this muscle loss is mostly due to lack of use. A decrease in muscle mass increases the risk of injuries, pain and degeneration. An increase in muscle mass can on the other hand decrease the risk for injuries, pain and degeneration.

A decrease in muscle mass and a increase in body fat equals a smaller motor in a bigger car. You will slowly hit shorter, play weaker, get a worse score, get weaker and feel older.

But you can do something about it…

Creeping Obesity

Creeping obesity is a consequence of a decreasing metabolic rate caused by less muscle mass and overeating. On average you will gain 15 pounds per decade or 45 pounds over 30 years and suddenly you will ask the mirror "who are you?" and "where did you come from?" The older you get the less muscle mass and the greater decrease in metabolic rate and increase in fat.

Decreased Mobility

A decrease in flexibility will affect your ability to perform the golf swing and your club head speed. Your flexibility is determined by your joints ability to move and dictates the safe ranges for your swing patterns. As you get older your flexibility decreases...

But you can do something about it...

Decreased Stability

Your balance relies on the feedback from your central nervous system, the eyes, inner ear and message receptors in the joints and soft tissues. To maintain appropriate spine position through your golf swing balance is really important. If you can not control your balance optimal during the swinging action, the golf swing will be compromised. As you get older the system that controls the balance becomes less effective...

But you can do something about it...

Decreased Power

Do you need to spend endless hours doing aerobic conditioning, such as running or riding bikes? No. But I am not here to bash aerobic exercise, but if you have a prober strength training program you will get a lot of aerobic effect while training your muscles and you will save time.

If you walk during a round of golf (I hope you walk whenever possible) it can leave you really tired on the last few holes. But playing golf is not the best way to increase you endurance.

If you make smart use of interval strength training and circuit body-weight exercises you can maintain strength and power and at the same time achieve amazing levels of cardiovascular fitness.

Learn More About to Improve Your Golf Game

Learn about how to fight chair-atrophy, improve mobility, stability and improve power in my online video training course.

http://www.plus40golf.com

How Does Aging, Biomarkers, and Strength Affect Your Golf

Remember this...we are all affected by age, easy-chair atrophy and creeping obesity...therefore fitness exercise should not only be about changing how the body looks, but to improve how the body moves.

Ten Factors are Associated with Aging

1. Muscle mass
2. Strength
3. Basal metabolic rate
4. Body fat percentage
5. Aerobic capacity
6. Blood-sugar tolerance
7. Cholesterol/HDL ratio
8. Blood pressure
9. Bone Density
10. Control of body temperature

This is What it Means for You

Factor (1) and (2) are directly related. When your strength increases your muscles grow and visa versa. If your strength decreases your muscles will wither. An increase in muscle-mass will elevate your (3) basal metabolic rate, but a decrease in muscle-mass will decrease your basal metabolic rate and you will gain weight - fat that is.

When your muscle mass increases (and you don't eat more) you will see a decline in (4) body fat percentage, but when your muscle-mass decreases you will see an incline in body-fat because of a decrease in metabolic rate. (5)

Aerobic capacity can increase by prober circuit oriented strength training without spending endless hours on the treadmill or the highway. If there is a decrease in muscle-mass there will also be a decrease in aerobic capacity. (6) A stronger, bigger muscle-mass is better at controlling your body's blood-sugar tolerance and thus a smaller muscle mass is worse at controlling your body's blood-sugar tolerance. (7)

Cholesterol/HDL ratio typically improves when doing proper strength training and when a decrease in body-fat percentage is seen, if on the other hand there is a decrease in muscle-mass and an increase in body-fat cholesterol/HDL ration typically worsen.

Strength training can also improve (8) blood pressure. (9) Strength training increases your bone density and lack of load and stress (easy-chair atrophy) can decrease your bone density (osteoporosis). (10)

And Lastly your body will be better at controlling body-temperature if it is top tuned, but worse at controlling body-temperature is in bad shape.

Surefire Pathway to Better Golf

There is a surefire pathway to hitting longer, score better, play better and feel stronger and younger. using correction exercise, strength training and a healthy diet.

But where do you start?

There are some important steps to take before starting the "Plus40Golf Academy" training program. Devoting the necessary attention to each step will make it easier to reach your goal.

Get Your Doctor's Permission

Before you begin the "Plus40Golf Academy" training program, be sure to your doctor knows you plan to modify both your eating habit and exercising habits. Show him or her this book, sp what is involved will be made clear. Your doctor will more than likely recommend a thorough physical examination, if you haven't had one in the last year.

It is easy to get overwhelmed, confused and suffer from analyse paralyse. That is why it is important to be honest with yourself and test your strength, endurance, mobility and stability to get an overview over your body ability and weak links.

How to Use Strength Training Exercises to Improve Your Golf Game

The primary effect of strength training is an increase in both the strength and the size of muscles. Strength training also affects in a positive way the bones, ligaments, and digestive and cardiovascular systems. Bodyweight exercises is also know as calisthenics (Greek words for beauty and strength).

You can choose between a lot of different strength programs. And you can choose between machine training, free weight training and body weight exercises. The all have pro and cons.

Why Do You As a Golfer Needs More Strength

This strength is the basis of all physical capability. It is what enables us to defy gravity and live life. Strength performs everyday tasks as getting out of bed, walk, run, eat and open doors. It is a fact that a stronger golfer is able to swing the club faster and hit the ball harder and farther and better control the muscles for more accuracy.

Most golfers spend a lot of money on the latest equipment and personal trainer sessions, but not much on their own physic, health and wellness. Imagine if you woke up tomorrow 25-50% stronger. Imagine how easy your everyday task would be and imagine how much easier a round of golf would be.

You will develop greater strength, reduce your body-fat level, improve your flexibility, balance & coordination and cardiovascular endurance.

How to Use Mobility Training to Improve Your Golf Game

What is mobility? Is it the same as flexibility?

Mobility refers to our ability to move freely without stress on the body. Our flexibility is dependent on the range of motion of our muscles. The two are not the same, but are not mutually exclusive. Good mobility can assist your flexibility and vice versa.

Is mobility more important as we get older?

It's important to be mobile at any age. The aging process can take its toll on the body, so it is important that we stay mobile and supple to combat this.

What are the main benefits of mobility training?

Mobility training can improve the range of motion of our joints and muscles. It can assist in improving our posture. Mobility training can alleviate 'everyday' aches and pains as well as improve our body awareness.

Is it ever too late to start mobility training? How soon could you begin to see results?

It is never too late to start mobility training. Your mobility is always something you can improve. In terms of results, this will initially be something you feel rather than see. You might feel a little less stiff after one or two sessions - but the key is to be consistent with your mobility training. Over time you should see an increase in your range of motion and perhaps improvement in your performance in other activities.

How to Use Stability to Improve Your Golf Game

Stability training refers to performing exercises while on an unstable surface with the goal of activating stabilizers and trunk muscles that may get neglected with other forms of training. Whether you're doing stability ball training or unilateral exercises like the ones in this workout, core strengthening is a surefire to prevent future back pain. Unilateral training, lifting weight on only one side at a time, prepares you for movements in daily living and sports that bilateral movements (using both limbs at the same time) may not cover.

Keep your core tight during full body stability workouts build to strengthning, preventing injury, and improving balance, coordination and performance.

Learn How to Test Your Mobility, Stability, Strength and Endurance

Learn more about testing yourself and how to use the test for improving yourself and your golf game in my online video training course.

http://www.plus40golf.com

Eat Right to Play Better Golf

Paleo Diet

The Paleo Diet has been called the caveman (or cavewoman diet, in this case) diet with good reason: it's based on the diet that our primal ancestors lived on back before wheat was harvested and there was a McDonald's in every town. While there are definitely cons to the Paleo Diet, there are also some health benefits to eating like humans did 10,000 years ago. The paleo diet definitely works for golfers as well.

Below are some benefits!

1 It's unprocessed. Simply put, caveman or cavewoman didn't have to worry about eating organic because everything was organic and natural without preservatives and artificial ingredients. Following the Paleo Diet helps you to eat a clean diet.

2. It reduces bloat. Want flatter abs? Reduce bloat by getting more fiber, drinking water and avoiding salt. All principles of the Paleo Diet!

3. It's high in fruits and vegetables. Besides protein, the majority of the Paleo Diet eating plan is made up of a diet rich in fruits and vegetables. Getting five a day in is no problem!

4. It's high in healthy fats. The Paleo Diet is high in omega-3 rich fish and nuts. These protein sources are full of healthy fats!

5. It's filling.

An other approach that works wonders alongside the paleo diet is intermittent fasting.

Intermittent Fasting

Intermittent fasting is not a diet, it's a pattern of eating. It's a way of scheduling your meals so that you get the most out of them. Intermittent fasting doesn't change what you eat, it changes when you eat.

Why is it worthwhile to change when you're eating?

Well, most notably, it's a great way to get lean without going on a crazy diet or cutting your calories down to nothing. In fact, most of the time you'll try to keep your calories the same when you start intermittent fasting. (Most people eat bigger meals during a shorter time frame.) Additionally, intermittent fasting is a good way to keep muscle mass on while getting lean.Improve Your Fitness - Improve your Game

Whether you want to hit longer, play stronger, score better or increase the numbers of years you are able to play golf, strength training should be the foundation of your conditioning.

The key to regain a strong, lean and healthy body that hit longer, play better, score better is to regain your strength, reduce your body-fat, improve your flexibility, improve your balance/coordination and your endurance through circuit strength training.

Learn How to Test Your Mobility, Stability, Strength and Endurance

Learn more about testing yourself and how to use the test for improving yourself and your golf game in my online video training course.

http://www.plus40golf.com

The Next Step, Are You Ready to Do Something About It?

What should an effective golf training program do? It should improve your golf performance and reduce the risk of injuries. But it should also improve your daily living. That is an increase in muscle-mass, decrease in body-fat, improved mobility, better stability and improved endurance.

25% of all recreational golfers experience back, hip, elbow and shoulder injuries that could have been prevented.

It should make perfect sense to you by now that golfers (especially over forty) can benefit greatly from a training program that conditions these vulnerable parts of the body.

The objective is to help you hit longer, score better, play stronger and to fight easy-chair atrophy and creeping obesity.

The Plus 40 Golf Academy program provides training programs that should help every golfer over 40, regardless handicap, fitness level and time constraints.

Frequently Asked Questions

Do you have a question? I have answered a lot of questions as a health-care provider! Maybe I have answered your question below! If not send me an email or tweed me.

Q: What is the "Plus 40 golf Academy Training" system and how does it work so well?

The Plus 40 Golf Academy system is a complete golf conditioning system designed specifically for golfers over 40 years of age. We cover workouts, diet and lifestyle and interview experts and players about how they do it in order for you to create a stronger, leaner and healthier body that performs better on the golf course and in you life. You will get stronger and feel younger.

There are fully detailed programs based on the level of fitness you are starting at. Everything is laid out for you in full detail. It is almost as good as having me guide you through it, every step of the way.

Q: What equipment do I need for this program? Can I do the workouts at home?

The workouts are designed to use bodyweight exercises only. But in certain situations you might need machines or free weights. This program has the advantage of making you proficient at using the one thing that you are never without: your body. You will get stronger, lose weight, improve your mobility, stability and power. Combined with a better nutrition and consistency you will be a totally new person and golfer. Workouts can be done anywhere, anytime and without costly gym memberships or equipment.

Q: How soon can I expect to see results?

Depending on your outset, you should notice results within the first 2 weeks. By the end of of your first month you should feel and see some noticeable changes on your physic and on the golf course.

Q: Do I have to spend countless hours in the gym or on the road every week?

Not at all. With "Plus 40 Golf Academy" system you will only have to train 2-4 times a week 20-40 minutes each time. The best of it you don't have to go to the gym. You can do it at home, in a hotel or where ever you are.

Q: Is this system only for advanced golfers?

No. There is different levels of workouts. Beginners, intermediate and advanced. Whatever level you're starting at, we have the program.

Q: I want to start today. How long do I have to wait for you to ship everything to me?

You don't have to wait! The entire "Plus 40 Golf Academy" system if online, you will get instant access to it as soon as your payment is accepted. There is no waiting at all. You can get started in the next 5 minutes. It is a ten week system and each week we will release a new module for ten weeks. We have experienced that if we released everything at once people felt overloaded.

Q: What if it doesn't work for me?

Then it is all FREE! No questions asked, 1 month money back guarantee, 100%!

I am so excited and believe so much in the benefits of this system that I am willing to let you try it all out risk-free for a full month. If you're not satisfied with the results and aren't completely excited with the system simply let me know and I'll give you all your money back. No questions, no hard feelings.

So test it out for a full month, experience the results for yourself and if it's not what you thought it would be I'll refund your money right away.

Note: "Plus 40 Golf Academy" system is an online membership site. No physical products will be shipped. After you order, you will get INSTANT ACCESS to the online membership site and all the bonuses from your computer. You can access the system from Mac or PC.

Who Am I and Why Should You Listen to Me?

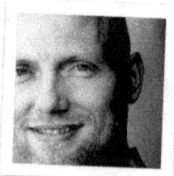 My name is Klaus Jørgensen and I have spent more than 12 years of my life as a Physical Therapist. I always wanted to eliminate pain and physical limitations by thorough precise diagnosis, targeted treatments and preventive measures.

More than 12 years of physical therapy has taught me that a lot of golfers suffers from easy-chair atrophy and creeping obesity, decreased mobility, stability and endurance.

Are You Ready to Do Something About It?

Introducing - PLUS 40 GOLF ACADEMY
Complete conditioning program.

The 10 week exercise program - transformation plan.

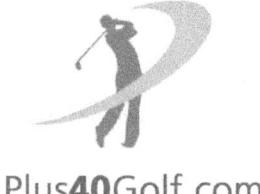

PLUS 40 GOLF ACADEMY is the program for the plus 40 year golfer who want to hit longer, score better, play stronger and who experience easy-chair atrophy and creeping obesity, decreased mobility, stability, strength and endurance.

The PLUS 40 GOLF ACADEMY complete conditioning program is packed with evaluation programs, different levels of exercise programs (beginner, intermediate and advanced programs), exercises shown on video, tricks, expert interviews, interviews with professional golfers about their training, nutrition and injury prevention, tips and advanced techniques that will help you get strong, lean and healthy to improve your game and your life.

No overly complicated scientific formula's or jargon that requires you to be a M.D in physiology or anatomy.

Just the truth about exactly what you have to do to hit longer, score better, play stronger, avoid easy-chair atrophy and creeping obesity.

If you are tired of back pain, injuries, feeling weaker every year, more overweight you need to take action and start applying PLUS 40 GOLF ACADEMY - the complete conditioning program and you will be surprise how much better you feel and perform on the golf course and in your life just 10 weeks from now.

Here is Just a Small Sample of the Discoveries You Will Find...

- How to evaluate your current strength levels.

- How to regain strength and muscles lost due to easy-chair atrophy.

- Why testing yourself matters the most.

- How to evaluate your current fat levels.

- How to get leaner and avoid creeping obesity.

- How to evaluate your mobility.

- How to improve mobility for a better golf swing.

- How to evaluate your current physical capacity level

- How to improve your physical capacity level.

- Interviews with coaches and professional golfers about their view on fitness for the golfer over 40.

- How to set yourself up for success

- What to eat and not to eat to avoid creeping obesity and to get a leaner more healthy body.

In Addition to the Core of the Course You Also Get...

Printable Workout sheets

You will get a fully detailed, step-by-step exercise beginner program. These workouts were designed with you, the golfer over 40 in mind and will fight easy-chair atrophy, creeping obesity, decreased mobility, stability, strength and endurance like nothing you have ever tried before.

The exact number of sets, repetition, rest periods are all shown to you on the simple and logical printable workout sheets.

All the guesswork and confusion has been removed. All you need to do is to follow the program for 8 weeks...Then go on the golf course, hitting longer, score better, feeling younger and stronger than ever.

Are you ready to do something about it...

Now is your time to get back into shape, hit longer, score better, play stronger, fight easy-chair atrophy and creeping obesity.

I'm giving you a full month to test drive the PLUS 40 GOLF ACADEMY Complete conditioning system - the evaluation program, the specific workouts, mobility programs...

And if at any point during the full month you are unsatisfied in any way, for any reason and don't think that PLUS 40 GOLF ACADEMY Complete conditioning system is the best golf conditioning system you've ever used, simply write me an email and I'll refund all you money right away...All of it.

That's how much I believe in this system.

See you on http://www.plus40golf.com

I can't wait to hear about your incredible results. Talk to you on the other side.

Kind regards,

Klaus Jørgensen
Founder Juviva Group and PLUS40GOLF
http://www.plus40golf.com

Hire Klaus Jørgensen To Speak at Your Next Event

Bring Klaus to your company, your conference, or your special event!

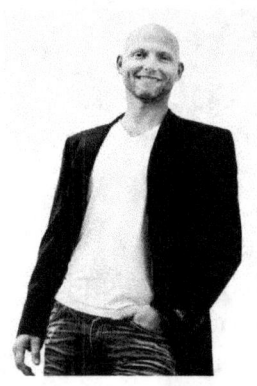 Klaus is an engaging speaker and his presentations are fresh and powerful. He has the ability quickly connect with his audience, gain their trust, understand their needs, and then guide them to new skills and understandings.

Klaus has developed the exciting and efficient "Plus40Golf Academy" designed to equip you as a golfer with the knowhow to pinpoint your weaknesses and correct them.

Please visit the http://www.plus40golf.com for more information about the "Plus40Golf Academy" and One-on-One Coaching

Speaking, Seminars & Coaching!

Bach. Physiotherapist
Cert. MDT
Cert. CMP
Cert. FMS
Cert. YBT

www.ingramcontent.com/pod-product-compliance
Lightning Source LLC
Chambersburg PA
CBHW071320280526
45788CB00004B/1963